Her Story

She didn't know when it would end ? She kind of knew that he was using her from the Get go, but, she couldn't prove it. Her life had taken a series of turns and acute angles. There was no telling when he was going to explode again.

She remembers very clearly what Sandra hd said when she was in jail, "We are all here for something." She was here for a reason. Looking back at that time in her life, she felt like experience had added more years to her life, rather than take them away. She was not going to quit trying. But for now, she waits.

She knew that on that particular day, not that long ago something was going to go down. She had been talking to this was had met online. She was going to see him that day and just say that she was going out to apply for jobs. She felt aggravated at the fact that her husband had been treating her as a dust collector, once again. She was also having a bad day with her medication for bipolar depression.

She only remembers that she ended up throwing a knife at her husband. It missed him, of course. He called the cops on her and she wound up behind bars.

This is her story.

The ride to the jail compound had been tearful and long. They had her checked in and she surrendered her phone and purse, first thing. Plastic bags were used to dispose of her belongings as she sat, cuffed, on the bench. She went in to the nurse's office as her name was called. She told them what meds she was on and for what diagnosis. She would later find out that she would have to have her husband bring her meds to drop off. She was issued orange scrubs and she couldn't wear her own bra. Orange crocs were given to her as well. The very first person made a phone call to was her mom. "You'll never guess where I am," she cried in the phone, "I bet you that I can..," her mom shot back. After the call, she was given a mesh bag with a plastic cup, spork and a blanket.

Then, an officer booked her in and led her down a long hallway where doors had scanners and buttons that they pushed, to enter and exit. F6 was the pod number that they stopped at. He opened the door and led her into an open room where 15 other ladies were seated on four metal tables, watching a tv show. There was a set a stairs that led to small cells above her. The officer led her to a cell on the bottom floor, straight ahead. Upon entering, there was a small metal table attached to the wall with seats, too. The bunk beds were on the opposite wall. Both were metal with a slim-looking mattress on top. "Your bunk is on top," said the officer. She took out her blanket that was rolled up inside her mesh bag and flung it on the top bunk. She precariously lifted herself onto the bed and spread out the blanket over the mattress. Her stomach growled. She hadn't eaten anything since breakfast that day and it was almost 6o'clock at night. She laid down and covered herself up. Locked up in a cell, alone with her thoughts.

So, this is what her husband went through a few years back. ..and all because of a damn roommate who he used to live with. She sighed. Closed her eyes and didnt open them again until an intercom woke her up early the next morning. It was coffee cake and hard boiled egg for breakfast. She ate it all up and carried her tray to the doorslot and set it down. Then, she climber back into her bed and fell asleep.

Later that day, her cell mate woke her up and asked if she was coming out to the table or staying in. J climbed down and put her crocs on, following her bunkee out to a table. There were 15 other ladies sittin down already. From what J could remember, her bunkee was Jessica from Norman, who was about four years younger than her and had a kid. Her bunkee had been b her about who she was and what she had done to be thrown in jail. She was in there for child endangerment and DUI. She had been in that jail for little over a year.

J felt that she needed to get to know more of the ladies in this place if she was going to be in there a while. At lunch, she sat across the table who went by the name of Amethyst. She was in jail for grand larceny and had been booked the same day as J was, apparently. The other lady sitting at their table was in there for "failure to appear in court". She went by the name Pam. She had been in there for little over a month.

The lunch menu was dried out spaghetti and an upside down cake with icing on the bottom. The drink was a lemon packet that she had to pour water & stirred up.

Another officer appeared to take the trays. About 30 minutes later, another was cme and it was time for "outdoor rec". J lined up with 7 others. She needed to breathe fresh air and get some sun while she could. Down the hallway they walked...until they stopped at a door that was marked "outdoor". Beyond the door, a wide area stretched beyond. Three brick walls surrounded the area and two cameras were facing opposite directions. The ladies stretched out on the concrete floor and laid out in the sun for 30 whole minutes.

Then, it was time to head out. She didnt want to leave. She had an idea as soon as she returned to her cell and asked her bunkee if she could borrow some soap and deoderant. She had noticed the weird looks from some of the ladies earlier. So, she took her towel and soap and headed for the upstairs shower. It was spacious and private, at least. And J enjoyed it! After her shower, she sat back down at her table and tried to focus on the tv show that was on the screen. An hour must have dragged by nd then another. Trays were delivered and they all had to line up single file. It was noodles with mystery meat and a cake for dessert. Yummy. She noticed that the food at this place was bland and badly needed salt. But there was no salt to be had, unless she had the money to order salt from the commissary. And commissary came on Tuesdays and Thursdays. She made a quick phone call to her dad and asked him if he could put $30 dollars on her books for hygiene products, paper, pencil and stamped envelopes.

She would make herself busy while she was in jail. She wouldn't be able to contact her hubby directly, but she would definitely communicate to him through her parents. Every day was the same routine. She usually slept in and skipped breakfast. She felt like she had already lost weight while in there. Her meds were brought to her bright and early in the morning. Mail arrived an hour before they went back to their cells. Her mom had sent her a postcard of a hummingbird and wrote, " Your hubby is not doing good. He's struggling to make ends meet." A certain panic started from there , yet there was nothing she could do but wait, praying for him.

Her arraignment was on the following Monday. She walked down to another room where there was a row of guys on one side, and a row of women on the opposite side. Once her name was called, she stood before a monitor. Her judge was LIVE and he spoke to her briefly about what she was in jail for. Assault and battery with a dangerous weapon. Her judge asked her to report back for her PHC in another week. They didnt call her name to go back though. On Wednesdays, it was laundry day. She had to line up with the other ladies and chunk the blankets and mattress sheets into a big bin, along with dirty underwear and socks taboot. After that, they sat back down at the tables and either played Spades or watched music videos. J wanted to learn how to play, so another lady, Sandra, taught her. J ended up learning from the best. She and Amethyst would team up against Pam and Sandra, then switch. They would play for two solid hours before it was time to eat or go to "indoor rec". Sandra actually braided J's hair! That was a treat and it looked cool. It took Sandra three hours to do it, though. Nothing happened on Thursdays except that J and her bunkee had cleaning duty first thing in the morning, right after breakfast. They had to sweep the open foyer area, around the tables, and in the bathrooms. Scrub the shower floors and then mop everything. J would climb back into bed and read the Bible or write. She kept to herself often enough, though her bunkee would rant about how long she was being offered to serve her sentence.

Twenty years in the pen. J would sit and listen, then offer some "out there" advice. For the most part, she enjoyed helping her bunkee keep a positive outlook on things. She was a mom, too. Yet, it seemed like every time she trned around, her bunkee would rant and rave about J's snoring and how little sleep she got. Which kind of pissed J off. She couldn't help it if her meds were causing her to snore. My, how attractive, by the way. Then Fridays would roll around and the book cart would appear. She loved selecting books. You could only pick two at a time. So, she found one and started reading it as soon as she got back to her cell. After lunch or toward the evening, she would join Pam and walk. They would walk side by side, back and forth, from one end of the stairway to past the upstairs shower was. At least 25 times. The following Monday, Sandra helped write out a few letters to find out who J's lawyer was and to the case manager to see if she would be added onto Mental Health court. Since both ladies figured that that was what happened to J and her husband, they could only try. Nobody wrote back, but J did get a hold of a psychiatric doctor, who wound up changing her meds a bit. They were limited in her mood stabilizer, so they had to do with what they had. They worked, though. She knew that as long as she kept taking her meds, she would not go ballistic or have any panic attacks after talking to her dad on the phone. Her dad, a pastor, told her that he wouldn't have anything to do with her husband or daughter because he felt that he was not the right person to help out, at that time. She flipped out and hung up on him! She ran back to her cell and cried her eyes out. All her fault. She didnt want her hubby and daughter to end up in a homeless shelter! But, what could she do? She cried herself to sleep that night. The next day, her lawyer called her back and wanted to meet with her. They had her line up with three other ladies, who also had conference visits. They walked back down the hallway and went through more doors. Then, they were told to take a seat outside a cubicle of rooms on one end of the hallway. It must've been 30 minutes before her name was called. She shook hands with a young looking fellow of about her hubby's height and the same age, too. He offered her a chair that sat across from where he was seated. She sat down, taking in her surroundings. "Well, Mrs. J, your husband called me yesterday and he had explained what happened. What I can offer you is five years' deferred with two years' supervision with a probation officer," he said. J looked down at the sheet of paper that she had to sign or not sign. She took a deep breath and sighed. She picked up the pen and signed her name on the dotted line, thinking things could be alot worse. She knew the three ring circus of the justice system. Always looking to make the poor man or woman pay more money out of pocket that they don't have. She thanked her lawyer for his time and then left to go back to her pod. Upon her return, Sandra asked her what kind of deal she was offered. J said, " Five years' deferred, two years' supervised." "That's more like it," exclaimed Sandra, holding up her hand to J for a high five. J went over to the phone and placed a call to her Dad to tell him what the lawyer had said. Her next court date wasn't until September 22nd; however, since her hubby had called ahead to have them switch her judge, she got in quicker. Her new court date was to be August 26th -early in the morning. It was a Thursday, so she had to live with one more weekend in this place. She continued to walk with Pam and confide in her annoyance at the justice system, some of the ladies in there, and the fact that she was ready to get out and move on in life! Pam was patient in listening to her thoughts and J was grateful that she had someone to vent to. One of the other ladies that had been shipped to rehab had written J back with her new address. J took out a piece of paper and wrote about what her lawyer had offered her and the fact that her hubby switched her judge to get her out sooner. Her bunkee offered J to do her eyebrows for her. She took a piece of thread from the lining of her orange scrubshirt and tied it in a knot. Then she twisted it to make it work like a set of tweezers. It was a little painful but nothing J couldn't tolerate. After her bunkee had finished, she looked ten times better. In the face, at least. She had about five sheets of paper left, so she went around to some of the ladies and offered to draw them a picture of their choice. One of them, she drew a rose; another, her name in calligraphy. She even wrote a poem called "Doesn't Hurt No More". Here's how it went:

So numb, so confused.

Why do I feel so used?

In jail, inside my cell...

I'm a dreamer

trapped inside a wishing well!

There is no pain

Everything is lost.

I'm inside a maze

But at what cost?

Don't know when, don't know how

but the feeling that I get...

is the brutal truth of the matter

that will be revealed yet.

So scared, so alone-it's like ice in my bone!

Help me, God, to be set free-

it's the real me...

that only You can see!

When she made another phone call to her mom, she found out that her hubby was all packed up and ready to take off for Colorado to go live with her youngest brother. She almost freaked out! So, she told her mom to tell him to go ahead without her, if anything. He would take their daughter with him, too. And she would be left behind. She didnt have anywhere to go or live?! But, with her court date set for that following Monday, it would be a close shave.

She would have to transfer her case to Colorado, if they were really moving there. She held her breath, and the weekend crawled by slowly until Monday morning finally arrived. The guard almost.yelled her name as she was just waking up from a fitful sleep. J asked the guard what time they would pull her to go to court. But, they didn't know, of course. So she made her bed up, got out a clean sheet of paper and drew a picture of a heart with angel wings. This design would be her trademark from then on. Breakfast was served ten minutes later. Malto meal, hard boiled egg and lemon drink mix. She shoveled that down and carried her tray to the doorslot. Then she climbed back onto her bunk and laid down for a few. It wasn't 30 minutes later that an officer called her to the open area. He had her face a wall outside the pod. Feet spread. Arms up. They scanned her legs, then arms. She was marched to the front desk and cuffed to another lady from another pod. They sat down in metalframed chairs for almost an hour. Then an officer came down the hall escorting ten guys that were cufflinked to each other. Another officer appeared out of thin air and lead her and the other lady into a small room the size of an elevator. They crammed all the guys in there, also, making it really jam packed. And hot. The first officer then led everyone out to where the vans were parked inside a bay area- off of the main front lobby area. It was kind of hard to maneuver into the van, what being cuffed to each other and all. But, they found seats and crammed all the guys and two girls into the vehicle. This would be the first time in over a month that she would be able to view the outer world. The streets went by as the van carried them to the downtown area. Not even fifteen minutes later, they were entering a gate behind a giant building. This would be the courthouse, she surmised. They parked in front of a garage door. The van doors opened, and everyone slowly exited the van onto the sidewalk. Then they followed each other, single file, through a doorway into a dilapidated looking lobby area. The paint was peeling big time all over the walls and the floors were dirty. They sat down on a concrete bench next the wall and waited for an officer to give them knew orders. Five minutes crawled by and there was no officer. Then a cop came in and dangled a bunch of keys that were attached to his beltloop. He unlocked the cuffs from the guys' legs first, then undid the womens'. J was the last. The officer then directed her and the other woman to a corridor that led to the left. Through more barred doors and into a very small open lounge area that had one metal table, a set of chairs, and a bathroom attached. There was graffiti all over the walls! She and the other lady took turns using the restroom and sat down at the table for what seemed like two hours or more. J got acquainted with this gal pretty easily although this one was headed for prison for possession of drugs. She still doesn't understand what the big deal is with drug laws and always wanders why they have to be illegal. It's the peoples' right and choice to use or abuse. She gets to thinking about all the money that the government would save the state- if the sale of marijuana was legalized. But, that was another topic. Finally, they were summoned to follow another cop. This time, they crammed into an elevator with the guys again. Ding Ding went the signal. The doors opened and they filed out into a broad hallway that opened up into two chambers. The chamber to the right was where they headed. In they went. There had to have been about ten lawyers present. And probably more within the next few minutes. The chamber opened up to a sanctuary type setting, where rows of pews, or benches, lined up.They went around the judge's podium and took a left after they passed the prosecutor's stand. They stepped onto a platform that held about thirty rotating chairs and took a seat, J at the very end, second row, next to a large window. More people filed through the doors. Briefcases scuffed the floors and papers shuffled like crazy. Then the judge entered with an "All rise". The judge looked at the people and replied, "Please be seated."   J was the first one called to stand up. "Good morning, Ms. ", greeted the judge, "You are charged with Assault and Battery with a dangerous weapon." She said, "Yes, sir!" " Your attorney and you have come forward today with the proposed deal that includes two year's supervised probation, five year's deferred sentence,"he continued. "Yes, sir!" The judge looked at her and said," Very good. Your next court date is set in four months time, in which you will not commit any said crime therein or forthwith...do you agree to this?"

"Yes,sir!" The judge shuffled some papers and then told her to be seated once more. Everything felt like a blur to her by the time noon rolled around and her stomach growled in protest, when finally, an officer reappeared to lead them back the way they came. She stood up and walked around the witness' stand and in front of the benches. She glanced over her shoulder and there was her husband. He smiled and mouthed, "Hey," to her. She turned her head then looked back and smiled at him. He had shaved his head completely! Wow! The last time she saw him was little over a month ago and she swore up and down that she wasnt going to talk to him ever again. But, now that things were looking up and she would be released soon enough. She lead the group, still cuffed to the arms, through another set of doors that faced another elevator. They headed back to the jail not an hour later. The ladies were separated from the guys as soon as their feet hit the ground inside the bay area. They went back in the same way they had exited before, only this time, they weren't shackled by the feet. An officer led them down the long and narrow hallway and through a door. A small concrete room with glass windows was their waiting area. A toilet was there for their use, but there was no privacy screen. Good grief. She and the other lady was issued a brown lunchbag that contained two bologna sandwiches, an orange, and a piece of carrot cake.No drink mix. Grr. They ate up their lunch and then their names were called. J was led back to her pod. Sandra exclaimed," What d'ya get?" J jumped onto the chair next to Sandra and said," Two year's supervised, five year's deferred! Will they release me today, you think?" Sandra finished shuffling her deck of cards and looked up and said, " Way to go....and yes, you will definitely be released today, sometime." J was so excited! But, three hours went by and there was no word yet. Getting a bit edgy at this waiting game, she walked some laps with Pam and told her everything the judge said. Then she heard her name being paged over the intercom. Things started to speed up again and the next thing she knew, she was being escorted out of the pod, saying a "goodbye" to all the ladies sitting behind her. With meshbag, blanket and spork in hand, she was led to the booking area. She made a quick phone call to her husband, saying " You wanna come and pick me up?" Her name was called and she hung up the phone. She handed in her meshbag, spork, cup and blanket. Then she was issued her outside clothes. Ahh, she thought, they smelled of cigarette smoke! Then they led her to the exit door...and not even a minute passed, when her daughter ran to her with open arms as she walked into the lobby area. Her husband smiled and offered her a cigarette. She drew in a deep breath and sighed. With relief. She was going home and she would NOT be coming back. Everyone was happy she was back. Life would start over for her and her family. To this day, J still wears her "jailhouse ring" that she created and placed on her pinky finger. Twas a reminder that she had a choice to make.

His Story

She thinks I have the damn key to the lockbox, but I don't have it, he said to himself. He had told her that, too. But she doesn't believe him! She was going on and on about how unhappy her life had become- then she turned around and gave him an evil stare. *She really hates me and I haven't done anything!* Was she losing her mind? Why did she want to get rid of him so bad? He felt disgusted. With himself and with her- his beloved wife of two and a half years. "*Are you trying to take me away from my own daughter?*" Maybe holding the kid as leverage would work. She answers back, " No, I am not." "Yes, you are!" She walks to the bedroom and slams the door behind her. He gets to packing. Packing what, he wasn't so sure. Most of this crap around the house was hers. He puts his computer stuff in a large box, bit by bit. She swings the door open five minutes later , carrying the lockbox in front of her. She's got a 'killer' look on her face. "You are not going to hit me with that, are you?," he dared to ask. She pauses briefly and squints her eyes, then goes into the kitchen. She asks me again," Can you pleeeeaaaasssse help me find the key?" "No." He wasn't going to give her the satisfaction of helping her out! The next thing he knew, he saw a piece of silver hurling through the air, coming towards him. It went past him and hit the wall with a clatter. She had thrown a knife at him! "You've lost your frickin' mind!" He stood up and grabbed her laptop that was sitting on her desk. He throws it at another wall and it busts into pieces before it hits the floor with a crash! He grabs the phone. She stomps over to the desk and picks up the knife and walks back to the kitchen, where she places it back in its drawer. He dials 9-1-1. "Yes..." "My wife just threw a knife at me and I need someone to come out here and help..."She listens and he talks to the operator, then she starts a crying fit, " You jackass! You really called the cops?" She stormed off again. He had their three year old daughter in his arms now. Shame that she had to see her daddy and mommy fight already! Then my wife runs up to the box that I was packing and starts throwing my computer stuff out the front door! She was mad with tears all over her face. This could NOT be happening! "You're only making this worse!" he blurted out to her. That only made things worse. She screamed at ,him, "Get the f*** out of my house!" A cop snuck around the corner, listening to all of this as she was still finding things to throw out. She stopped her rampage as soon the cop spoke up. He didn't want their daughter seeing what might happen next, so he walked down to the pool area with their daughter. Then there were two more cops going into the house. Wtf?? They escorted her outside to a wall and sat her down. Then a cop approached him and asked what had happened. He told him that she needed to get some help. Not jail. However, twenty minutes later, they were leading her out, handcuffed, to a squad car. He couldn't believe what was happening! What in the world had she said to them? And what was he going to do now? He had a lot of phone calls to make. He called her mom first. Maybe she could help out or something. Not five minutes later, I hung up the phone feeling frustrated and betrayed. Her mom just told me to go to a homeless shelter. And with my daughter, too! That is no place for a three year old! So I called my wife's brother who was in Colorado. "Something has happened to J?," her brother guessed as he picked up the phone. "Yes. Your sister is in jail." Silence. Then her brother said, " I will be there in a few weeks. That's all I can do for now to help out." "Okay," he replied, holding his daughter close. Little did he know that in calling the cops in the first place would set their housing on the line. For the next three weeks, he called the D.A. and her lawyer to find out when her court dates were. He also had to switch her judge to get an earlier hearing date. That took forever. And they had raised her bond to $20K because they failed to pull her for her court appearance. At home, he was a full-time single dad now. Things were getting worse for his daughter ,too, as she was getting crankier and crankier. He finally ended up taking his daughter to the emergency room to find out what was wrong with her. They said that she was constipated and had head lice. Great. So he was prescribed some medication for both and took her home.

Never would he envision the pains it would take to get rid of the lice in her hair. But voila! Twenty minutes later, the process was done and he could lay her down for bedtime. He decided to write his wife a letter. He had some ideas as to what he wanted out of their relationship now that he had the time to think about it. They had been through too much to just give up now. He wouldn't be able to give the letter to her until she was released from jail. It would have to wait. Oh, if only he knew if she still loved him enough to work together on their marriage..?? He had no idea. The next day, his best buddy called and asked how things were going. He told his buddy what had happened. The buddy went off on a rant about how lousy his wife was for doing that. He should've stuck up for her better. But, things were looking bad anyway. He made a few phone calls and got a hold of her lawyer. According to the lawyer, the bond was set at $10,000. And she was looking at being charged with a felony because the state had picked it up. His daughter wasn't looking too well either...now what?! His daughter was crying at night more and more, holding her tummy. He decided he would take her to the emergency room to see what was wrong with her. They checked her vitals and took her temperature. All normal. They laid her back onto the bed and felt her tummy. She cried out. The doc looks up at him and says that she is constipated, altogether writing out a prescription. "Oh, by the way...your daughter also has lice." He sighed a heavy sigh and went by the pharmacy for the prescription. He took his daughter home and debugged her hair twice, using all the medicated lotion that was prescribed. The next day, a lady and a man from the local DHS came knocked on the door. He was fearful that they had come to take away his daughter because of what happened. However, they just came by to ask him a few questions about what happened and to see if he needed any help with anything. "I don't know how to go about putting her in Headstart?" he asked after a few minutes of thinking. They gave him the paperwork and referred him to a school so he could go ahead and get her enrolled for the Fall. He called her lawyer once they left. And that's when shit hit the fan.... They had raised her bond to $20,000 for a bench warrant. "But, she was in custody this whole time! He said to himself. He needed to find out who her judge was going to be and try to talk to him about this whole mess. He was used to this three ring circus of a justice system. He was going to get her out of jail some way! He awoke with a start. He had heard sirens going off. He felt panicked and his heart was racing! He ran to his daughter's bedroom and peeked in. She was playing with her Barbie dolls quietly. OK...he thought, she is safe. He missed his wife. No such thing as a good sleep since she left. He felt miserable and fell into an endless and soulless routine in caring for his daughter and making another round of phone calls to help his wife get released. Her court date was coming up the following Monday. So, he showed up at the courthouse expecting to see her and that's when he found out that she wasn't going to be released until two months later. Sheez! He didn't know what to do? He took his chances on an idea. He dialed a number and let the phone ring four times. "Hello?", said the voice on the other end. "Yes, something has come up and to make a long story short, your sister is in jail." Silence and then, "What happened?" "Your sister lost her mind and threw a knife at me." "Why did she do that?" "We were fighting over a key to the safe box and she just snapped." "I'll be right there in a couple of days... I have to work the rest of my shift and then I will drive down there to help out." "Okay," he said and hung up the phone. He had no idea if he could hang in there for another few days..!? The phone rang and the caller ID displayed a DETENTION CENTER. He picked it up..."Hello?" And it was her. His wife. But how? Then he knew how without even asking. "How are you doing?," she asked. "Not good. Our daughter won't eat and she had lice." "I'm so sorry. Poor girl. Just wanted to check up on you myself." He didn't know how to respond nor did he know what to say. "Don't have a lot to say right now...I am trying to get you out of there..."he continued. "Okay. Hope things get better soon. Love and hugs," she said, then the phone went silent. He put his daughter down for a nap and he laid down on the couch, but couldn't sleep. His mind wouldn't stop racing. All his problems and all of his worries were taking a toll on his body and mind. She had the nerve to call him! So, she must still care... he just didn't know how much. He got up and went online and listed some items to sell. He would make some money in the process. There was another knock on the door. This time it was a woman with a briefcase. "Can I help you?" "I am Kim. I am from Human Services Outreach...I needed to collect some information about your case." "Ok..", he held the door open for her. "How are things going?" "Right now, things are okay. Had to buy a bunch of lice medicine for my daughter's hair." "Okay..."she said as she made some notes on a notepad. "How is your daughter doing otherwise?" "She misses her mom, but me and her, well, we're doing okay." She scribbled more notes. "Do you know that your daughter can qualify for Headstart for free?" "No, ma'am, I didn't know." "Well, allow me to dig in my briefcase here and get us started on the process!" "Okay...", he said as he scratched his chin. He wasn't good at asking questions like his wife was or, for this matter, Miss Kim. "Fill these worksheets out as best you can and then give them back to me when you're finished. Do you have any questions for me?" He looked up at her and said, "Probably not the kind of questions that you deal with..." She glanced at her watch, then closed her briefcase. "Then I will be back in a few days to get those papers from you." After she had left, he placed a call to the District Attorney. He had to let someone know the whole story behind his wifes' situation. After twenty minutes talking to the D.A. ,he realized he was getting nowhere. So, he turned around and called her indigent lawyer. The answer came all too easily. He had to ask to switch her judge...so that his wife's court date would be sooner than the original court date. Thirty minutes later, the deed was done. He woke his daughter up from her nap and played with her til suppertime. He called his father in law to see if he had talked to his wife anymore. She had. And she told her dad that she still loves him...even though they both agreed on the fact that he calling the cops, was the wrong thing to do. The phone rang as soon as he hung it up on its cradle..."Hello?" "Hey, moron! What's happening? Is she still in the clink?" "Yes.." "Do you still love her after what she did to you??" "Yes, I do." "why?" "Why not? Her meds weren't working that day. We got into a fight...et cetera." "Man, I hear ya...but I am a little pissed off at her...glad she's not my wife!" He hung up the phone on his "friend" from Washington. There would always be drama with that guy. And he wasn't putting up with the insults about his wife. She wasn't really a violent person!

August 26th rolled around. Today was the day his wife had court. He had her brother at the house, watching his daughter, while he went to the courthouse. He got there right as the officers were seating the detainees. He found her on the top row at the very end. Damn! She lost weight. The judge came in on an "all rise"; then, they called her name first. She stood up, obviously handcuffed to the other lady on the same row. "You are here today because you are charged with Assault and Battery with a Dangerous weapon." Yes, sir," she replied. " You agreed to the punishment of 2 years supervised probation, five years' deferred." "Yes, sir." "I expect you to keep up on your fines and all your domestic violence classes until they are finished. I will see you in 120 days." "Yes, sir," she complied with no expression. Then she looked right at him! He mouthed the word, "hey" to her. An hour later, the judge was finished with the majority of the list and the officers summoned the detainees to follow them out the courthouse doors. She passed right by him. She sneaked a glance and an "I love you", then went out the door. Time flew by that day. He went back home. He was restless. She should be getting out today. She should be getting out today! He cleaned the house and made the bed... not that he slept on it these past 39 days. It was the couch for him! Then the phone rang. It was her! "You ready to come get me?" "Yes." He got himself and their daughter loaded up and drove to the detention center. The lobby was spacious with lots of chairs. He and his daughter sat down and waited. Twenty minutes later, she came through the door, all smiles. First thing, their daughter ran to her momma. Lots of love and hugs for the three of them. Then his wife said the famous last words, " I need a cigarette!" Oh, how he missed her!

Ecclesiastes 3:1 For everything there is a season, a time for every activity under heaven.

Epilogue

6 months later.

It was a cold and rainy day in hell. She woke up feeling angry again. Just like the day she threw the knife...only worse. She felt like hurting herself. Hurting others. She knew that she needed help. Fast. She turned to her hubby and said," Honey, I need to go get some help." He took her word for it and drove her and her brother (who came along) to the Emergency room at the local hospital. Once she was checked in, the hospital staff assigned a security officer to her room. They gave her a gown and a blanket to change into after she deposited her clothes into a blue bag. She was there for three hours before a pair of cops came to escort her, in cuffs, to their car. They drove her to a mental hospital about thirty minutes away from home. The cops dropped her off at the reception area, where she was admitted. Five minutes later, she was introduced to an Admission specialist, whom she had to fill out an endless array of paperwork explaining why she was there. Then she was lead to a nurse's station where they gave her a pair of socks in exchange for her shoes. Laces were considered contraband. As were bra under wires. No belts and no drawstrings from hoodies or pants were permitted. They lead her to a room that serviced two single wide beds. Hers would be closest to the window, looking out over a field of grass. She sat down on her bed and drew up the blanket around her shoulders, taking in her new home surroundings. She dropped the blanket a few minutes later and walked to the day room area where there were other people sitting on couches and chairs in a large semi-circle, facing the tv overhead. A nurse handed her a styrofoam carton that contained a burger with ruffled chips and was accompanied by a bottle of Sprite. She sat herself down in one of the chairs along the far north wall. "Is that a burger you're eating?", asked a lady who was sitting opposite her. " Yes," was her reply. That lady would easily annoy the crap out of her if it wasn't for the fact that she was being watched closely. That night would be the longest night of her life. She laid there looking up at the ceiling, tears streaming down her cheeks. Nothing mattered, she thought. There would be tomorrow but even then, that was no guarantee. A voice woke her up out of a groggy state of sleep. It was a nurse asking if I wanted breakfast. Crap. She knew it was still early because the sky outside her window was dark. She mumbled a "No thank you, " then went back to sleep. She finally woke up when the nurse came back, asking her if she was going to have lunch. She sat up in bed and rubbed her eyes. What time was it, anyway? Time to get a watch, she muttered under her breath. Lunch consisted of a Chicken Club sandwich with ruffled potato chips and a gatorade. She scarfed down her meal and went to sit out in the lobby area where the tv was blasting out some music videos. She fixed herself a cup of coffee, then crossed over to the far wall, again, to sit in her usual spot. The doctor motioned to her with his hand to walk over to where he was standing. She obeyed. "You doing okay? How are you?" Great. This was an eastern indian guy with an accent. "Fine. Just been sleeping a lot." "I put you on Zyprexa, Lithium, Fluoxetine, and Ambien. Today you get your blood drawn from nurse, ok?" "Okay." It would be the same routine all day every day for the next week and a half. She woke up on a Sunday thinking it was time to try to go home. She was feeling better. She wasn't sleeping all the time now. But for some unknown reason, that same doctor would not let her go home just yet. Each morning, it was the same things...blood pressure check, meds check, breakfast, and then group therapy, where everyone had to participate. The tech people asked them what goals they have for that day,and the people would tell them. Then, it was 'do your own thing' for the next hour before lunch would roll around. She figured out the timing of her calling home right after she finished lunch around 11:30 a.m. Things would be rough at home. Her daughter would be testing her dad's limit on various things. Typical four year old drama. Then it was time to either watch t.v. or go to your room. She chose to go back to her room. She would read her book or play Sudoku, in which she had to hide her half a pencil in her folder. That would be considered contraband as well as hardback books. She had already pulled a naughty note in sharing an e-cigarette with another lady that was a bit of a rebel. That was fun.

Then her name would be called to see her therapist. She put it out there that she wanted to go home, however, her therapist could only recommend her release per paperwork. So, she got a stress ball out of the deal anyways. After talking with her therapist, she filed a grievance against her doctor, for not letting her go home. Suppertime came around and then visiting hours commenced! Her dad was the first guest to see her. She told him what all she was doing to fill her days with. Same shit, different day. But the best timing was right after her dad left, her hubby showed up along with her brother and brother-in-law. Her brother(s) looked at her in sympathy and told her that they missed their SkipBo challenge. She told them that she was working on getting released. Her hubby missed her terribly. Their daughter was doing great in school still, but she was asking where Mommy was at, off and on. That gave her heart a pang of fierce love. How much she missed her kids! Her Uncle Jo and Aunt Margaret came to visit the next day. At the very end of their visitation, Uncle Jo handed her a few booklets. "Just a little something for you to read while you're in here," he said to her. She went back to her room to read the booklets. "And Peter.." was the name of the first one. And she ended up liking that one the best because even though the Apostle Peter denied Christ three times, Jesus still called upon the disciples ....and Peter. It was a great source of encouragement even though she was not a religious person. Not much happened that made a profound impact on her a few days later. The doctor still wouldn't release her. So she waited patiently for Tuesday to roll around. Tuesday was "court" day, in which the patients' had the right to go in front of a judge and get the 'override' to be released. The judge was the only one that could go above the doctor's word. It snowed! She watched the snow fall endlessly and peacefully outside of her window. Man, the patients weren't even allowed to go outside! At least she was able to request a nicotine patch up in here. Yes, she was a smoker. And her next goal upon getting out of there was to quit smoking for good. She walked back and forth down the hallway for four to five times. Then she stopped at the window that was at the end of the hall. It was still snowing, and she was stuck in here. Where was the REAL help when it was needed? She started to cry. Sorrow for not being strong. Sorrow for missing her kids. And sorrow that after all these terrible things that happened last year, this is what it came down to. Betty snuck up on her. Betty was the biker chick that was a room down from hers. "You're going to get out of here soon." "I hope so." Sniffles. She and Betty walked a couple of rounds down the hallway. Then the nurse called for Betty to get her things from her room. "Ain't that some shit," said Betty, they hugged and parted ways. Story of her life. All of her friends were either out of town or out of state. No sense making friends up in this joint! She fixed herself another cup of coffee and sat down in one of the chairs in the lobby area. The lady, who spoke to everyone, was rather quiet today. She let an inward sigh of relief. She wasn't in the mood to talk to anyone. She didn't understand why she was here except that she had a nervous breakdown, and felt like slapping the crap out of people. She didn't feel like that anymore though. But, she needed to get to the bottom of her anger issues. Yes, she was angry at her mom for divorcing her dad. Yes, she was angry that her mom was remarrying a biker dude. Yes, she missed her grandma very much... her grandma had passed away a year ago. Then she lost her maternal grandma six months after that. Then she was tossed in jail for throwing a knife at her hubby. No, this was not a good year. She even lost a younger cousin to kidney failure. All of these issues came down her so fast, she became paralyzed with anger and depression. In dealing with these issues, she had not allowed herself to grieve properly. She was expected to keep her wits about her. She was the oldest grown kid. But, she felt so lost and she realized that she didn't know her "illness" anymore. IT was hard figuring out where she stood on when it came down to her relationship with her mom. Her relationship with her dad wasn't as close as she wanted it to be. Some things were better left on the shelf. Jerking back to the present, she barely heard her name being called at the nurse's station. The admission lady summoned her to the double doors. She followed the lady into another hallway. They passed by at least five doors, then they made a right. She was lead into a small room where the 'lawyer' sat at a table with a chair and a security officer looked on. The lawyer made her sign her name on a few sheets of paper, then lead her to another room where there was a long table and four people were seated as if they owned the place. They looked over her case and within two minutes, made their decision. She was free to go home. !!!! She could barely believe her luck! She skipped back down the hall to the double doors that lead to the "psych ward". She waltzed back to her room and started gathering her things. The nurse found her and gave her her medications, then took her blood pressure. Normal. She asked the nurse if she could use the phone to call her hubby to come pick her up. Woo Hoo! This place was depressing and she knew that once she left, she would start to perk up a bit. She knew that the first thing she would do was get out her computer and start writing all about this venture. It was a long two hours before her hubby showed up. Oh, but how glad she was to see him! She walked up to him and gave him a hug. Things were going to have to change for the better. They just had to.

"And ye shall know the truth. And the truth shall make you free." John 8:32

This book is dedicated to

My entire family...whose love

Knows no boundaries.

www.ingramcontent.com/pod-product-compliance
Lightning Source LLC
Chambersburg PA
CBHW081203280526
45787CB00008B/3385